The Legitimate Diet

Timothy Scharold MD

- Smart

    No complicated menus or rules
    A choice of plans to fit your needs
    Set your own goals
    Puts your body to work for you

- Easy

    No unreasonable limits
    Eat food you like
    Gentle phase-in period
    Full of practical tips

- Physician designed

    Safe and reliable
    Proven results
    Scientifically sound
    Uses your natural bodily mechanisms

Legitimate Diet

The Legitimate Diet

Timothy Scharold MD

Legitimate Diet

Legitimate Diet

Contents

APPENDIX

Other Top Ten Tips

About the Author

Dr. Timothy Scharold is board certified in Internal Medicine and Geriatrics and has additional training in diabetes, cholesterol, and hypertension. Throughout his 20 plus years of practicing medicine, he has dealt daily with the results of unhealthy diets. As he found himself spending a lot of time discussing his patients' bad cholesterol and glucose levels and advising them on strategies for improvement, he decided to search for simple resources that would help them improve their diets, and thus their health. But, most of the information that already existed was confusing, complicated, and unhelpful. So, he created his own manual that distills the basics for healthy eating into one simple plan. This book is a result of his years of reading and teaching about healthy eating and weight management. And now, included in this new edition, are Dr. Tim's Top Ten Tips!

For more diet information,
Visit: www.LegitimateDiet.com.

A special thanks goes to my daughter Kristen Scharold for her invaluable input.

All information provided in this document is based on the opinion of the author. As always, the reader should clear any dietary changes or supplements with his or her own physician.

"Let food be your medicine and medicine be your food."
— Hippocrates, 400BC

Introduction

How are you doing? How are you feeling about your diet? Your weight? Your health? Your energy level? Your well-being? We all think we should feel better, and think we can do better. Wouldn't you love to be thinner, feel better, and have more energy? Our limitations are usually a result of our bad habits, lack of motivation, and perceived inability to change. Most of this stems from life long habits, wrong assumptions, and a confusing mass of miss-information. Even if you want to figure out what is best for you, finding out how can be overwhelming. Before the Internet, I was astounded at how many diet books existed with confusing information. Library shelves were overflowing with them! Now thanks to the Internet, this confusion has been multiplied to unprecedented levels.

You have more control over your health and weight than you may realize. I have seen in my twenty plus years of practice, that most health issues arise from poor diets. Actually, they are more like toxic diets. I am sure you have heard of the obesity and diabetic epidemic in America. This is a result of our diets, which are often driven by our natural desire to eat, our impulsive habits, our lack of self-control, and the ease of getting whatever we want when we want it. Advertisers have been more than happy to drive our diets and supply us with what we want to the detriment of our health. If you, or anyone, desire to be healthy now and in the future, and not be dependent on health care to keep you going, it all begins with an improved healthy diet now! But where do you start? Well, you can start right here with this book.

To correct any problem, first you need to figure out the cause, and then fix it. For example, if your car is not running properly, you need to figure out what's wrong before you can repair it. Throughout this book I will compare our body to an engine. You will be amazed at the similarities. You will discover how important quality food, a.k.a. our fuel, is to have a well-running body. So I will begin by explaining the many problems in our diets and then I will show you the "easy fix." You can become your own health maintenance mechanic.

This book will be your guide in the basics of what you need to know to have a well-running body. You will learn not only how to *eat* healthy but also how to *be* healthy. And as an added bonus, I'm sure you will lose weight, which can make you even healthier.

PART ONE

Healthy Foods
High Quality Food for Fuel

TOXIC AMERICAN DIET

Americans seem to be drawn to a toxic American diet. This is a diet that is highly processed, calorie dense, and nutrient depleted. It not only makes us fat, but also endangers our health. A toxic diet (and obesity) leads to hypertension, diabetes, high cholesterol, cancer risk, gallbladder disease, sleep apnea, and arthritis.

The toxic diet is mainly from highly processed foods. They are readily available in grocery stores or at fast-food restaurants. They are advertised to get you to consume them. They tend to contain excessive amounts of unhealthy fats, refined sugar, sodium, and preservatives. This is why they can be made cheaply, taste good, and last a long, long time. Example: Twinkies have been known to never spoil. Margarine can last indefinitely even after opened.

YOUR BODY: A LEAN MACHINE

Your body is an energy machine. We all have driven a car, or at least traveled in one. And we know it's not fun when it breaks down. The car essentially becomes useless, unable to do what it is meant to do. Similarly, our body can break down, posing potentially life-threatening risks. But, prevention with good maintenance and quality fuel is the key to avoid catastrophes. Any machine will run better, last longer, and is less likely to break down when properly maintained, treated well, and supplied with the best fuel.

Just as an engine runs better and gets more miles per gallon with high quality fuel, your body works better with fewer calories if they are quality calories. Quality foods are more satisfying to your body and turn off your hunger drive while allowing your body to function longer without needing more fuel. Plus, it is less likely to store the fuel (in the form of fat) if it burns it well.

If your machine runs smoothly, it will last longer and not need as many repairs. Furthermore, your body will be able to better handle the demand and stress placed on it. When a machine runs on bad fuel it not only produces a bad smell, it releases more toxins and pollutants that affect the machine itself. Over time this eventually can cause the engine to break down. There maybe cheaper fuel, but it won't burn as well, and in the end, with the damage it causes, it does not save any money and does more harm than good. The same is true with your body so it's time to be smart about what you put into it.

Quality Foods

Enjoy and thrive on a low quantity of high quality foods.

Quality foods contain all three-food groups: carbohydrates, proteins, and fats. You naturally desire all these because your body uses them in different ways. Your body can even convert one food type into the other. This converting takes energy, so your body prefers to have all three raw materials supplied in food. When your body is supplied with all three food types, it turns off the "feed-me" drive sooner.

Let me give an example. Have you craved something sweet after a meal? Do you feel more satisfied with pie or ice cream? That's because the combination of carbohydrates and fats, after protein consumption, turns off the hunger drive and releases endorphins (endogenous narcotics) which signal satisfaction. Unfortunately, that tends to lead to us to eating more of the desserts and sweets. The trick is to limit the amount by eating it slowly and savoring it, thus giving the feedback mechanism time to kick in. It usually only takes a tablespoon size of dessert to accomplish this, not a huge serving or two.

CARBOHYDRATES

Glucose

Glucose (sugar) is the essence of all carbohydrates. Glucose is our body's engine's essential fuel. It is needed for muscles to contract (including your heart muscle), and supplies energy for your organs to do their great variety of work. Our brains are so picky about glucose that they function only with pure glucose as a source of energy.

Our body breaks everything down to this basic element so it can use it for all energy processes. This carbohydrate breakdown, or digestion, begins in the mouth with our saliva, and continues in the gut. It breaks the complex carbohydrates (chains of sugar) into the basic glucose element. That is why if you chew bread long enough, it begins to taste sweat in your mouth as the glucose molecules are released. This can explain why bread and pasta are as enjoyable and addictive as candy and other sweets are to eat.

Too much sugar can overload the body, like too much fuel can flood an engine, causing it to lose power and waste energy. Too little sugar can make you tired at first. But the body has an amazing ability to convert fat and protein to glucose when needed. That's one thing an inanimate machine cannot do. The conversion process can go the other way too. When your body has had enough sugar, it will begin storing it up AS FAT. As long as you burn all the carbohydrates, there should be none leftover to produce fat. And, the only way the fat will be used is when there is not enough sugar available.

About 60% of our diet is made up of carbohydrates, some good, some bad. Reduce the bad carbs and you can improve your heath, and reduce your weight. It is as simple as that.

Sugar and Flour (The White Stuff)

Sugar and flower make up most of our carbohydrate intake. These are useful purely for energy and have no nutritional value otherwise. These are the extra calories that are the cause of our obesity epidemic. *Reducing these useless carbohydrates calories is the easiest and most obvious way to reduce weight.* Flour is typically made from highly processed wheat. Recently authors have come up with a book called *Wheat Belly*. In this book they describe the ravages and pit falls to our poor health which they say is a result of our wheat and flour obsession. In another book, *The Carbohydrate Addict*, doctors describe the same problems and dangers of carb "overdosing." These sugars are so addictive because of the crazy carb cycle described below.

Starches

Starches (bread, pasta, potatoes, and rice) are also carbohydrates, essentially a calorie source. These are considered more complex, because they need to be broken down into the sugar molecules before use. They may have some nutritional value. They are basically fillers. Cutting back or eliminating these from your diet can make a big difference in your weight. Most people love one or the other of these starches (usually pasta or bread). If you're going to consume the pasta or bread, you are better off with high fiber brands (whole wheat bread), eating them with other quality foods (proteins), and limiting the portions.

Junk Food
Junk food is typically carbohydrates with bad fats (candy, desserts, and crunchy snacks). These may satisfy the taste buds, but not the hunger drive for long. It is the worst culprit for the crazy carb cycle, which just makes you hungrier.

The Crazy Carb Cycle

The crazy carb cycle is the quick rise and fall of sugar levels in your blood stream. Most flours and sugars are highly processed. As a result, they are quickly absorbed and quickly raise your sugar level. A sudden rise in the sugar level causes a large release of insulin. The sugar level then drops quickly while the insulin level remains high. The dropping sugar levels and high insulin levels stimulate the "Feed me, I need more fuel!" drive. As a result, snacking on these highly processed foods (junk food) creates a vicious cycle of over eating. This is a serious problem for dieting. *The cycle must be stopped or no diet will work.*

Insulin Resistance

Insulin resistance occurs when the cells stop responding to insulin as a result of this vicious carb cycle. Insulin resistance can lead to diabetes. Furthermore, the high insulin levels result in more storage of carbohydrates as fat, which also increases the risk for diabetes. High insulin levels also increase LDL, the bad cholesterol, and lower HDL, the good cholesterol. The cycle goes on and on. Studies are starting to show that high insulin levels may be one of our greatest health risks for obesity and heart disease.

The Metabolic Syndrome

The metabolic syndrome is another bad result of this carbohydrate over load. People with metabolic syndrome have some or all of the following: high blood glucose, high blood pressure, abdominal obesity, low HDL elevated cholesterol, and high triglycerides. This is a result of developing insulin resistance, and is a precursor to diabetes. It is also found to be a risk factor

> ***Dr Tim's Top Ten Tips***
> **#1**
> **Eat Less White Stuff.**
> Eat two less servings of the white stuff each day.

for heart disease. It is the basis of morbidity from our obesity endemic.

Everyday I counsel patients on the problems of the metabolic syndrome. Just looking at the lab tests, I can see if they have been enjoying their American carbohydrate overload. I can also tell by looking at these numbers weather they have really reduced those dreaded carbs or not. The good news is that more people are listening and changing their habits.

Glycemic Index

The glycemic index is a measure of how fast carbohydrates raise the serum glucose level. It is compared to pure sugar, which has a glycemic index of 100. The high glycemic index foods, by raising glucose levels quickly, cause the carb cycle of highs and lows discussed above.

Three factors that reduce speed of entry of glucose into the blood stream are the amount of fiber and fat in the carbohydrate and the complexity of the carbohydrate. These result in a lower glycemic index. Most vegetables, fruits, beans, and grains have a low glycemic index, whereas white bread, white rice, potatoes, pretzels, and refined corn have a high glycemic index.

Ten Worst Glycemic Index Foods

White Bread, French fries, cookies, breakfast cereals, potato chips, baked potatoes, whole milk, Ice cream, chocolate bars, soft drinks, and juices.

Complex Carbohydrates

Fruits and Vegetables

Fruits and vegetables are the best source for good carbohydrates. They contain natural fiber that limits their quick absorption so you do not have the insulin surges resulting in high serum sugar levels. Scientific studies repeatedly find diets high in fruits and vegetables (high fiber) result in many health benefits and longevity.

Fruits and vegetables contain many vitamins and minerals that are good for your health. These include vitamins A (beta-carotene), C, E, magnesium, zinc, folic acid and phosphorous. Scientific research repeatedly shows fruits and vegetables can fight against all types of diseases. Vegetables and fruit contain phytochemicals, which are 'plant chemicals.' These biologically active substances can help reduce your risk of:

> *Dr Tim's Top Ten Tips*
> **#2**
> **Eat More Fruit.**
> Have at least one extra fruit and veggie each day.

- Diabetes
- Strokes
- Heart (cardiovascular) disease
- Cancer – some forms of cancer, later in life
- High blood pressure (hypertension)

Fruits and vegetables are low in fat, salt and sugar and provide a good source of dietary fiber. A high intake of fruit and vegetables can help:
• Reduce obesity and maintain a healthy weight
• Lower your cholesterol
• Lower your blood pressure.

Fruits and vegetable are high in fiber, which has many health benefits discussed later in this book. These fiber help slow sugar absorption and reduces cholesterol absorption, helping control sugar blood levels and cholesterol. All this results in a reduction of heart disease, stroke, and diabetes.

Fruits and vegetable are very high in antioxidants, which are thought to be another source of the health benefits discussed above. Read below for more on antioxidants.

Best and Worst Carbohydrate Foods

Ten Best Carbohydrate Foods: Blackberries, Blueberries, Raspberries, Strawberries, Cauliflower, Broccoli, Kale, Lettuce (darker green the better), Spinach, Apples.

The Worst Carbohydrate Foods: sugar, potatoes, rice, bread, pasta, cookies, candy, ice cream, pies, and muffins.

FAT

What are fats? There are many different types of fats. Our body needs certain fats to function normally. They are very important in cell walls. Fats also make a great storage of energy. 9 calories per gram is double the calories in protein or carbohydrates. Imagine having twice as much fluffy fat than what you currently have as storage. Our body uses fat as a back up survival mechanism. This storing of energy as fat is a major difference from our engine model we have compared the body to. That's why engines are always lean machines. You may wish you did not have this storage mechanism, but then you would need to be eating continuously.

Two Types of Fats: Bad and Good

1. Saturated fats: These are more solid at room temperature, and mostly from animals, such as red meat and milk products. They are not good for you. Super-saturated fats and trans fatty acids last forever, are man made, and found in packaged foods like cookies, chips, and pastries. These are the really bad ones.

2. Unsaturated fats: polyunsaturated and monounsaturated fats. These tend to be liquid, and are usually from plants, such as vegetable oil and fish oil. These are the good fats.

The Bad Fats

Saturated Fats and Trans Fatty Acids: These toxic fats raise bad cholesterol levels, increase risk of heart disease, Alzheimer's disease, diabetes, and cancer.

Saturated Fats

Saturated fats are animal fats, such as red meat, butter, milk, and cheese. These are more natural unprocessed fats. In high doses they are not good for you. But low to moderate consumption may not be so bad. They are usually associated with good proteins. So it can be ok to eat a little at a time. If consumed in moderation, they may not be harmful.

Trans Fats

Trans fatty acids are the most toxic of the saturated fats. They are manufactured fats, from vegetable oils, that are supersaturated by a process called hydrogenation. This gives the food prepared with them a long shelf life. Foods with Trans Fats include: cup cakes, candy, chips, cookies, crackers, doughnuts, margarine, french fries, and vegetable shorting. They are cheap and last long, making it very profitable to produce and sell, but at the cost of your health. Studies show that a diet high in Trans fatty acids doubles your risk of dying from coronary heart disease.

Top Ten Trans Fat Foods
The worst stuff for you.

1. Spreads: margarine, shortening, butter.
2. French fries, or anything else fried.
3. Frozen foods: pies, potpies, waffles, and pizza.
4. Cake and cake mixes.
5. Cookies, especially prepackaged.
6. Chips, any kind that are packaged.
7. Crackers, except maybe some new "no trans fat, high fiber" ones.
8. Breakfast foods: doughnuts, pop tarts, danishes, etc.
9. Candy: gummy bears, jellybeans, etc.
10. Toppings and dips: creamers, gravy, bean dips, etc.

Red Meats

Red meats are high in saturated fats, and trans fatty acids. Red meats include beef, pork, and all processed meats (like: salami, hot dogs, bologna, sausage, bacon, etc.). Research repeatedly shows an increased risk not just for heart disease, but also cancers (colon, breast, prostate, and pancreas), diabetes, hypertension, and premature death. Not only are red meats high in

> *Dr Tim's Top Ten Tips*
> **#3**
> **Eat less meat.**
> Give up the red meats.
> Not more than one serving a week.

bad fats, cooking it generates cancer-causing compounds, like oxidants, heterocyclic amines, and nitrosamines. The more well done the meat, the worse the toxins.

Red meats have omega 6 fatty acids that tend to promote inflammation in the body, which has been found to be associated with multiple health problems. More on inflammation later.

The NIH, after extensive research, has found a very clear "association between red meat and increased risk of mortality." But, diets high in fish, chicken, and turkey showed a decreased risk of death. Several other studies show an increase of heart attacks by 30% from high red meat diets. On the positive side: heart attacks have been reduced by as much as 30% when red meat was substituted with fish, poultry, or nuts in daily diets.

Best and Worst Fat Foods

Ten Best Fat Foods: olive oil, macadamia nuts, almonds, avocados, pecans, cashews, flax seed, salmon, herring, and canola oil.

The Worst Fat Foods: Vegetable oil, margarine, red meats (ground beef, sausage, bacon), liver, hot dogs, bologna, chips, pies, cakes, cookies, candy, doughnuts.

The Good Fats
Unsaturated and Omega-3 fatty acids

Unsaturated fats: These are fats that are not "saturated" with hydrogen ions. Polyunsatured fats are even better. These are liquid oils, mostly from plants and fish. They have been found to reduce cholesterol levels and reduce heart disease.

Olive oil is an excellent example of a good unsaturated fat. It is the backbone fat of the famous Mediterranean Diet that has been found to be so healthy. Its use can lower LDL (bad) cholesterol, and has beneficial anti-inflammatory, antioxidant, and anti-thrombotic properties. Olive oil has also been found to help with weight loss, particularly sustained weight loss.

Omega 3 Fatty Acids

Omega 3 fatty acids are polyunsaturated fats that your body needs but cannot produce. We can now measure omega-3 levels, and studies are showing up to 90% of Americans are deficient in omega-3 fatty acids. Omega-3 deficiency can lead to and increase allergies, arthritis, asthma, cancer, depression, diabetes, heart disease, hypertension, and sudden death. Some studies suggest that omega 3s have anti-inflammatory benefit, with a reduction in aches and joint pains. I like to think of Omega 3s as "oiling" your engine to keep it running smooth.

Omega 3s are in high concentration in fish and certain

25

cooking oils (olive oil, safflower, sunflower, walnut, hazelnut, and almond oil). Use these oils whenever given the chance. Fish oil is an excellent source of the omega-3s. Cold water fish, like salmon and herring, have a particularly high concentration of omega 3s. Most fish have some level of omega 3s, making all seafood an excellent healthy food choice.

Fish oil

Fish Oils, or Omega 3 fatty acid supplements, are a great alternative for those who dislike fish, or don't care to eat three servings a week of salmon. Studies show that taking 2 grams of fish oil a day is equal to eating two serving of salmon per week. One study found that daily intake of fish oil reduced the risk for heart attacks by 25%, and may help to slow aging. Other studies suggest it helps neurological function, perhaps even help prevent Alzheimer's. It also has lots of vitamin E. Some experts recommend up to 10 grams of fish oil a day.

Dr Tim's Top Ten Tips
#4
Eat more fish.
Have a serving of seafood
or fish oil everyday.

Cholesterol: A Very Important Fat

Cholesterol is a soft, waxy substance found among the lipids (fats) in the bloodstream and in all your body's cells. It's an important part of a healthy body because it's used to form cell membranes, some hormones, and it is needed for other functions. But a high level of cholesterol in the blood—hypercholesterolemia—is a major risk factor for coronary heart disease, which leads to heart attacks.

Cholesterol and other fats can't dissolve in the blood. They have to be transported to and from the cells by special carriers called lipoproteins. There are low-density lipoprotein (LDL) and high-density lipoprotein (HDL).

LDL cholesterol: The BAD Cholesterol.

Low-density lipoprotein is the major cholesterol carrier in the blood. LDL cholesterol, as it circulates in the blood, can slowly build up plaque in the walls of the arteries feeding the heart and brain. This plaque can clog arteries and cause clots to form.

The latest research on bad cholesterol: Health science has advanced enough that we can learn more useful details about what makes the LDL so bad. The research has been motivated by the fact that 50% of heart attacks and sudden death occur in patients who have "normal" cholesterol or "normal" LDL. Now we are able to break the LDL down into sub particle measurements that tell more details of the pathological process leading to atherosclerosis, heart attacks, and strokes. The new measurements include the following:

Non HDL Cholesterol: The total bad cholesterol includes LDL plus other bad particles including VLDL, IDL, triglycerides and chylomicrons. This may be a better measurement of risk than LDL alone.

LDL-P (number of particles) and sdLDL (small and dense particles): It is the small particles that are able to get in the artery walls and cause all the trouble. The more there are the higher the risk of trouble. Thanks to magnetic resonance we can quantitate the number and size of your LDL particles.

Problematic lipid proteins—LPa and ApoB. LPa: is a protein that helps the LDL attach to the artery wall. ApoB is a protein on the LDL that allows particles to enter the artery wall.

How do these LDL particles and proteins cause trouble? Essentially the more of the smaller LDLs, with the bad proteins ApoB and LPa, the more they get stuck in the artery wall, causing irritation and inflammation. White cells attack the plaque, causing oxidation of molecules and even more inflammation. This leads to plaque build-up, which over time can rupture, causing a sudden blockage of an artery. In the heart that would cause a heart attack, or in the brain it would cause a stroke.

What can I do about the bad LDL particles? A healthy diet and exercise as outlined in this book are the first line of defense. There are also supplements and medications that can help. All options should be discussed with your health care provider. Hopefully this will add to your understanding of your health and motivate you to follow through with a legitimate healthy diet.

HDL cholesterol: The Good Cholesterol

HDL carries about one-third of blood cholesterol. Medical experts think HDL tends to carry cholesterol away from the arteries and back to the liver, where it is passed from the body. HDL removes excess cholesterol from plaques and thus slows their growth. HDL cholesterol is known as good cholesterol because a high HDL level seems to protect against heart attacks. The opposite is also true: a low HDL level (less than 40 mg/dL in men; less than 50 mg/dL in women) indicates a greater risk. A low HDL cholesterol level also may raise the risk of a stroke.

Dr Tim's Top Ten Tips **#5** **Eat more nuts.**

How does my diet affect my cholesterol?

Common sense would suggest that if we eat less fat, then our cholesterol should improve. That was the thinking of the experts in the 1990s. However a maverick physician by the name of Adkins, found that carbohydrates were a major problem, not just the fat. Here is how it works: If you eat more fat, your body breaks it down as it digests it, which takes energy, and the body tends to use it as it needs it rather that store it as fat. On the other hand, if you eat more carbohydrates, all the extra carbs you don't burn off get converted to triglycerides. The triglycerides are either stored as fat or converted to cholesterol. So you see, if you eat a low-fat but high-carbohydrate diet you will likely end up fatter with a higher cholesterol level. Since the 1990s "low fat, high carbs craze," Americans are fatter than ever, and the consequences of high cholesterol are out of control. This legitimate diet can help.

Ten Best Cholesterol Lowering Foods

Almonds, beans, cinnamon, flaxseed, high fiber fruits and vegetables, oatmeal, soy nuts, whole grains, and cold-water fish: salmon, tuna, sardines.

PROTEIN

Protein is the best of the three types of food because it has less calories, absorbs slowly, stops the insulin rise and fall, and supplies your body with important building blocks. There seems to be no bad proteins out there.

Protein is an important component of every cell in the body. Hair and nails are mostly made of protein. Your body uses protein to build and repair tissues. You also use protein to make enzymes, hormones, and other body chemicals. Protein is an important building block of bones, muscles, cartilage, skin, and blood.

It takes energy to break down the proteins you eat, and then your body builds them back up. This is how muscles are built. Exercise will stimulate this assimilation of protein into your muscles. As a result, the protein you eat tends to not be used for energy or stored as fat.

Studies have found that just increasing your protein intake (not fat) has resulted in early satiety, less calories-consumed, increased fat-burning, and weight loss. Higher protein diets are associated with lowered cholesterol, decreased risk of diabetes, and fewer heart problems.

Protein Sources: The best protein sources are those with limited fat, such as the plant proteins found in nuts, beans, whole grains, whey, and soy.

31

Meats are a high source of protein but they tend to have a lot of fat with them, especially the red meats. An ounce of almonds has as much protein as an ounce of rib eye steak. The leanest meats are seafood. Shellfish are the lowest in fat, even though what fat they have is cholesterol, your body breaks that down and uses it too, rather than creating more cholesterol. Fish, especially salmon, are an excellent source of protein, and the fat they have is of high quality: omega 3 fatty acids. (see below).

Poultry are the next leanest meat if eaten without the skin. Turkey is the next leanest. White meat is lower in fat.

Eggs are an excellent source of protein, The egg white is excellent and full of protein, and

> *Dr Tim's Top Ten Tips*
> **#6**
> **Eat more eggs.**
> Don't worry about the yolk.

even the yolk has been found to be good for you in spite of its limited cholesterol.

Milk products also have protein, but only the skim milks are low in the bad fats, and they still have some sugar in them too. Low fat Greek yogurt is a good option for dairy protein.

Snacks: Nuts, beef jerky, pork skins, and protein bars make a good protein snack.

Top Ten Protein Foods

Ten Best Protein Foods: Fish (especially, salmon, cod, mackerel, sardines, bass, tuna), shellfish (especially crab, lobster, scallops), eggs, skim milk, turkey, chicken, nuts, beans, whole grains, and soy.

The Worst Protein Foods: They are highly processes, with lots of trans fats: ground beef, sausage, bacon, baloney, hot dogs, salami, peperoni, lamb, and pork .

Diet Factors Affecting Your Health

Before we get into the legitimate diet details, I would like to go over other important points of a good healthy diet. These include the concerns of inflammation, free radicals, and vitamins and minerals. All of these are important for your health and they are greatly affected by you diet.

Inflammation

Inflammation is a condition where the body attacks what it thinks is harmful. The result is release of various byproducts that end up causing further harm. This can and does occur anywhere in the body, including the arteries that supply important blood to organs, like the heart and brain. Researchers are finding that a chronic condition of inflammation can harm the whole body. One of the common byproducts are oxidants, that end up damaging and aging the cells. Over time, repeated damage to cells can cause anything from rapid aging and heart attacks or stroke from plaque rupture, to damaged organs that do not function as well.

This inflammatory process is what researchers consider to be a major cause of aging. One study showed men with low-grade inflammation performed worse on standardized intelligence tests and were more likely to die from a premature death.

We now have ways of measuring inflammation, so we can do something before it is too late. hs-CRP and lp-PLA2 are two important markers. If one is elevated, research has found a 5-fold increased risk of a stroke. If both are elevated there is an 11-fold increased risk of a stoke.

Foods such as red meats and high processed food tend to release more toxins that cause inflammation. Also, don't forget about the small LDL particles that get into the artery walls causing inflammation. Another source is high elevations of insulin, from high carbohydrate intake, which has also has been found to aggravate inflammation.

Scientists have demonstrated how high fat levels in the blood stream cause inflammatory reactants to be released in the artery walls within 30 minutes of a fatty meal. These inhibit the release of nitric oxide (a chemical that helps dilatation of arteries), which causes arteries to constrict, leading to decreased blood flow, which can cause clots to forms, resulting in heart attacks. This was shown in volunteers who ate a burger and fries and then within 30 minutes, had the significant spasms or constrictions of their arteries. This could explain why there seems to be an increase in heart attacks during the super bowl.

Being overweight is another cause for chronic inflammation. Adipose cells release inflammatory proteins into the bloodstream, resulting in a chronic state of inflammation. Arthritis and chronic infections have been found to do the same. Periodontal disease can also raise inflammation levels. Several studies found chronic periodontal disease as a risk factor for heart disease and early death. Food additives and exposures to toxic chemicals and pollution have also been found to raise the levels of inflammation.

Dr Tim's Top Ten Tips
How To Stop Inflammation
1. No fast foods
2. No red meat.
3. Eat more anti-inflammatory foods (see below)
4. Take your vitamins (and other antioxidants)
5. Exercise reduces inflammatory levels.
6. Loose weight with less fat, helps: thin people have less inflammation.
7. Drink lots of water to flush out the toxins.
8. Fish oil has been found to be anti-inflammatory.
9. Aspirin is the ultimate anti-inflammatory, with anti clotting benefits too.
10. Lipid-lowering medications like statins lower inflammation that build plaque in your arteries.

Oxidation

Free Radicals: Free Radicals are molecules that are short of one electron, and they will do what ever they can to get one from other molecules. When they steal other molecule electrons, it is called oxidation. Oxidation, the loss of electrons, is now recognized as a major cause of many health problems, from heart attacks to early aging. The oxidation causes cell damage, that leads the body to see the cells or molecules as a foreign invader, causing our immune system to react, resulting in inflammation. The inflammation can lead to plaque buildup and artery clogging. The free radicals have been found to damage DNA in cells causing them to age quicker, or even change into cancerous cells. Free radicals can damage all body systems over time. They are considered to be "the biggest impediment to your quality of life."

Free radicals form from toxin exposure, like pollution or smoking. Free radicals also are produced from food digestion. More free radicals are produced from "toxic" foods. For example, highly processed foods, when digested, leads to the free radical production and release into the blood stream. Red meats, especially ones that are over cooked, have been shown to produce significant free radicals as well. Overall, just eating too much food can produce too many free radicals. Studies have shown that animals and people who consume fewer calories live longer.

Free radical oxidative stress can be measured by testing

myeloperoxidase levels. It is an enzyme that is released by the white cells when they are fighting "foreign invaders."

What can be done to stop these deadly free radicals? Fortunately, there are good foods that can help offset the damage (oxidation) caused by the free radicals. They are known as antioxidants.

Antioxidants have extra electrons that they can give to the greedy free radicals, without causing any harm (oxidation) to themselves. This saves the other cells from being damaged. Antioxidants are proving to be a lifesaver for every cell in our body, organs, muscles, joints, and brains. They are our main protective agent in the aging process as well.

As you can see, the more antioxidants we consume, as opposed to oxidizing foods, the better off we are. So what are the better antioxidant foods? That's easy: fruits and vegetables. They are full of the vitamins and minerals that are antioxidants. By the way, the more colorful they are, the more anti-oxidation power they tend to have.

Top Ten Antioxidants
by Color

Color	Source	Antioxidant
1. Orange:	Oranges	vitamin C
	Carrots	vitamin A
2. Red:	Tomatoes	vitamin C, lycopene
	Beets	pectin,
	Apples	quercetin
3. Green:	Grapes	resveratrol; very potent
		gives wine its health benefits
4. Blue:	Blueberries	flavonoids, anthocyanin, vit. E
5. Green:	Broccoli	carbinol, sulforaphane
	Asparagus	folate, glutathione
	Tea	catachins.
6. Dark Green:	Kale, Spinach	beta-carotene, lutein, flavonoids
7. Yellow:	Garlic	allicin, dially disulphide
8. White:	Cauliflower	glucosinolates, quercetin
	Radishes	quercetin, sulforaphane
9. Purple:	Pomegranate	ellagitannins.
10. Brown:	Coffee and Tea	catachins, polyphenols, flavonol, anthocyanidin, methylpyridinium

-**Spinach, kale, and broccoli** are vegetables with the highest anti-oxidative capacity.

-**Berries: blue, black and red**, are fruits with the highest anti-oxidative capacity.

Vitamins and Minerals

Vitamins: The molecules essential to body functions that our bodies are unable to make. We must get them from out side sources like food or supplements.

Vitamin A (Beta-Carotene), carotenoids, powerful anti-oxidants. In most fruits and vegetables, especially broccoli, spinach, kale, and berries.

Vitamin B- 1,2,3: Important role in energy metabolism. Found in some whole grains, and a lot in protein: meat, fish, poultry, and dairy products.

Vitamin B-6: Niacin. B6 is critical for protein and fatty acid metabolism It can lower LDL, and raise HDL. It is found in whole grains, but 98% gets processed or milled out. Also high levels are found in soybeans, poultry, beef, pork, and fish, especially tuna and salmon. Niacin has been used as a supplement to treat hyperlipidemias.

Vitamin B-12: critical for neurological function and lowering homocysteine levels. Only found in animal products: like fish and red meat.

Vitamin C: also known as ascorbic acid, is essential for repair of all body tissues and involved in many body functions, including formation of collagen, absorption of iron, the immune system, wound healing, and the maintenance of cartilage, bones, and teeth. Plus it is a very power antioxidant. It is abundant in fruits and vegetables, but not in grains.

Vitamin D: Essential for bone structure and cartilage, which includes heart and blood vessels. A lot of recent research has found up to 50% of Americans deficient in Vitamin D. Vitamin D is essential for many critical body functions. Low levels of vitamin D have been associated with everything from an increase in colds to an increase in heart attacks and premature death. Vitamin D comes only 30% from our own production, requiring sunshine. Food sources are vitamin D fortified dairy products, and fatty fish: salmon, sardines, and mackerel.

Ten Benefits of Vitamin D

Vitamin D reduces colds, diabetes, atherosclerosis, hypertension, heart disease, stroke, breast cancer, Alzheimer's disease, kidney failure, depression, tooth cavities, and food allergies, and osteoporosis.

Vitamin E: A very potent anti-oxidant and anti-inflammatory. Vitamin E is important in maintaining healthy nerves (memory), and cardiovascular system. Best sources are seed oils and fish oils.

Vitamin F: Ok there is no vitamin F, but let's just call it FRUIT. As we have discussed, you should be able to see how fruits are essential to us as they are chocked full of the essential vitamins we need. And a big part of their benefit is the antioxidant qualities, which can offset much of the free radical production from our toxic American diet.

Do I Need Vitamins?

In the past, well-rounded meals provided us with the vitamins and minerals we needed. But today's food is grown in nutrient depleted soil where only fertilizers are used. This, in turn, is fed to the animals, which are then injected with hormones to make them grow fast. As a result, most of our food today is deficient of the vitamins and minerals we need. Thus, I recommend everyone take a multivitamin with minerals and phytonutrients daily. Think of them as a safety blanket for your good health as you age.

MINERALS: I will mention a few important ones. Generally they are found in fruits and vegetables and some grains, yet a multivitamin with minerals may be your most reliable source.

Calcium: Helps bones and nervous system. Found in dairy products, and broccoli, kale, spinach. Needed to help maintain bone structure, along with Vitamin D.

Chromium: helps regulate insulin levels by improving insulin efficiency. Found in meat, cheese, legumes, and soybeans.

Magnesium: Involved in over 300 enzymatic reactions, especially cardiovascular metabolic processes. It lowers blood pressure, stabilizes heart rhythms, and reduces risk of heart attack and stroke. Found in nuts and green vegetables.

Molybdenum is an element that is present in very small amounts in the body. It is involved in many important biological processes, including function of the nervous system, the kidneys, and energy production in cells. Molybdenum is an antioxidant that appears to prevent cancer by protecting cells from free radicals.

Potassium: important in nerve conduction and muscles contraction. Seems to help with muscle cramping too. Like magnesium, it lowers blood pressure, stabilizes heart rhythms, and reduces risk of heart attack and stroke. High levels are found in avocados, broccoli, and citrus fruits.

Selenium: Is needed for the enzyme glutathione peroxidase that plays a key role in neutralizing free radicals. Many studies suggest it has anti-cancer benefits. Found in seafood, meat, and beans and nuts. Less in fruits and vegetables (except spinach).

Zinc: Important in maintaining a healthy immune system. Often used to fight colds. Some studies suggest benefit with memory. Best source is beef, chicken and seafood.

> *Dr Tim's Top Ten Tips*
> *#7*
> *Take a multi vitamin*
> *with minerals daily.*

Other Important Supplements. Supplements fall under the category of "food product" according to the FDA. The discussion of supplements could take a whole book, and is a confusing and controversial area of research, with inconsistent scientific proof of benefit. I will focus on the few that I believe may actually be beneficial.

Cinnamon: found to stimulate the efficiency of insulin, helping to stabilize sugar levels and diabetes. Other studies suggest a benefit in lower blood pressure.

Co Q10: Coenzyme Q10 is needed in every cell of the body. Your body makes CoQ10, and your cells use it to produce the energy your body needs for cell growth and maintenance. It also functions as an antioxidant. Levels are particularly high in organ meats such as heart, liver, and kidney, as well as beef, soy oil, sardines, mackerel, and peanuts. CoQ10 can help protect the heart and skeletal muscles. It is found to help in muscle and joint pain, especially aches that sometimes occur with statin use, and improves energy.

Pepper: Black pepper contains peperine that has been found to curb the appetite, decrease fat levels in blood, and decrease the formation of new fat cells. Chili peppers have capsaicin that cause sweating, raises your metabolism, releases the "feel good" endorphins in the brain, and helps relieve pain. They also are high in the antioxidants vitamin A and C, and have been found to lower cholesterol levels. And they do not in reality cause ulcers; they just irritate the heck out of them.

Phytonutrients

Other important nutrients found in foods that can benefit you are known as phytonutrients. Phytonutrients are plant foods that contain thousands of natural chemicals or phytochemicals. These chemicals help protect plants from germs, fungi, bugs, and other threats. They can help protect you from ravages of aging: including oxidation, inflammation, and cancer. Phytonutrients aren't essential for keeping you alive, but when you eat or drink phytonutrients, they may help prevent disease and keep your body working properly.

Fruits and vegetables contain phytonutrients. Other plant-based foods also contain phytonutrients, such as: whole grains, nuts, beans, and tea. More than 25,000 phytonutrients are found in plant foods. Some important phytonutrients are carotenoids, ellagic acid, flavonoids, resveratrol, and glucosinolates. These phytogens give the green, yellow, orange, and red colors to fruits and vegetables.

Carotenoids act as antioxidants in your body, they tackle harmful free radicals that damage tissues throughout your body. They are plentiful in greens such as: spinach, kale, and collards.

Ellagic acid is found in strawberries, raspberries, and pomegranates; and may help protect against cancer through several different ways. For example, it may cause cancer cells to die. And it may help your liver neutralize cancer-causing chemicals in your system.

Resveratrol is found in: grapes, grape juice, red wine. It acts as an antioxidant and anti-inflammatory. Some research suggests that resveratrol might reduce the risk of heart disease and cancer. And it may help extend people's life span.

Glucosinolates are found in cruciferous vegetables, including: brussels sprouts, cabbage, kale, and broccoli. The glucosinolates turn into other chemicals during the cooking process and while you digest these foods. These chemicals may help hold in check the development and growth of cancer.

Source: Web MD

Vinegar: for Early Satiety and Weight Loss.

Apple cider vinegar, the most popular, is acidic and contains vitamins, mineral salts, and amino acids. Two teaspoons daily have been used for good health since ancient times. There are a lot of medical uses of vinegar that have no scientific proof behind them. However, there are a few studies that suggest a true benefit. Vinegar may help diabetes by reducing glucose levels. Small studies show that it may lower cholesterol levels, lower blood pressure, and kill cancer cells. If nothing more, vinegar can help you feel full and reduce weight. Use it when cooking, on your salad, or with cucumbers (pickles), if you don't want to drink it straight down.

PART TWO

Principles of Dieting

Who made it so complicated?

Perhaps you're reading this to learn how to lose weight. You will learn that, but you will learn more. You'll learn a better, healthier way of living. In reality, "dieting" is something we all do every day. In general, a diet is what we eat. Today it is known as an attempt to eat less and lose weight.

Most diets are unsuccessful because we resist "dieting." We naturally want food and our bodies will store any excess. Our bodies are very efficient machines.

Have you dieted in the past? Did you lose weight? How long did it stay off? Why don't diets work? Are they too extreme or too complicated? Do they have unrealistic goals or are they hard to stick with? Are they based on unsound information?

There are three essential characteristics of successful diet:

1. Tolerable. In order to lose weight, a diet needs to be simple to live with. You shouldn't have to measure foods, read long books, or eliminate all your favorite foods.

2. Do-able. Most "experts" make dieting too complicated. Libraries are overflowing with books on dieting; most are complicated, confusing, and bogged down in detail. The Internet, the new information source, is even more overwhelming. A good diet must be easy to follow, using common foods that are easy to get and taste good.

3. Durable. If you are motivated to make the effort to shed those extra pounds, you want to be sure they don't find you again. You need at diet that you will be able to live with the rest of your life, not just a quick intolerable fix.

After many years of discussing weight loss and its benefits with patients and trying different methods myself, I have tried to design what I think is the best program for everyone. Of course for this to work, it will mean a change in how you eat, what you eat, and how you exercise. The reality is, if you do not change your eating habits, you are not going to change your weight.

Are you are ready to make a change?

Obesity: Your Motivation to Lose Weight

- Obesity contributes to over 300,000 deaths a year.
- It costs $100 billion annually in medical expenses.
- It contributes to many medical illnesses including diabetes, hypertension, stroke, heart disease, arthritis, some cancers, and sleep apnea.
- The average person gains 2% of their body weight each year.
- Since 1999, over 50% of the U.S. population is overweight (greater than 20% of their ideal weight).
- Just losing 10% of your weight can improve all the above problems.

The Legitimate Diet will help you to lose weight without the common struggles. It's something you can live with and enjoy. You will be able to lose weight and keep it off. It will help you look and feel better. Plus, you will be healthier for it.

The healthiest and most effective weight loss is only 1-2 pounds a week. It is consistency in your diet that is essential. If you are not sure how much you should lose, refer to this chart.

Ideal Body Weight

How much should you weigh? There are many complicated formulas, percentages, and tables, but none are as easy as the simple one below. It is based on insurance industry standards for evaluating health risks based on weight. Ideally, you should weigh less than the listed weight for your height.

	Weight (in pounds)	
Height	Men	Women
5'0"	130	125
5'2"	140	135
5'4"	150	145
5'6"	160	155
5'8"	170	165
5'10"	180	175
6'0"	190	185
6'2"	200	195

- BMI (Body Mass Index) is another measurement that takes into account your height and bone mass. It has become the new standard. The formula is:

$$(\text{Weight in pounds}/(\text{height in inches})^2) \times 703$$

- Some scales can estimate this for you. You can also use an Internet calculator. A BMI greater than 25 and you are considered over weight. A BMI over 30 and your are considered obese.

-The above numbers calculate a BMI of about 25.

-If you weigh 30 pounds more than the reported weight in the chart above, you are considered obese, or 20% over ideal weight with a BMI greater than 30.

CALORIES-IN VS. CALORIES-OUT

Your Body: The Energy Machine

Think of your body as a very efficient machine. It takes energy or fuel to keep you going. As a warm-blooded animal, you need to keep that fire burning. Without fuel, your "fire" dies out. As long as you are alive, you are always burning some fuel. This fuel is food, which is measured in calories.

Calories

Calories are a measure of energy based on heat. A calorie is defined as energy needed to raise one kilogram of water (about a quart) one degree centigrade. A calorie is basically the amount of heat or energy given off when food is burned.

You burn on average about 1500-1800 calories a day. These are the calories-out. You burn 1000-1200 if you are doing nothing but lying in bed. How much you burn depends on your metabolism or activity level. You can increase calories-out to 2400+ a day, with an increase in activity (e.g. exercise or increase in metabolic rate).

Your body can be compared to a furnace, as discussed earlier, with one exception. If you over-supply a furnace, it just burns hotter and hotter. But, if you over supply your body, it stores that extra fuel in the form of fat. Your body is amazingly efficient. Its natural instinct is to save whatever excess fuel it receives so it can draw on these reserves whenever needed. It is a wonderful survival plan, just not convenient in today's society of food abundance.

Your body stores this energy in a *condensed* form: fat. Fat has twice the calories (energy) as protein or carbohydrates. Fat stores 3,600 calories per pound! So you do not need as much space per pound for the energy stored. Imagine what we would look like if our fat was twice the volume and fluffier. You see, fat can be good for you if it's not in excess.

Alcohol

Alcoholic beverages are carbohydrate drinks too. They require a different method of burning fuel, which creates bad by-products. These do not provide any nutritional benefit, and make your brain and muscles function poorly (in case you never noticed).

Hard liquor on the rocks has the lowest carbs. The sweet mixers are the problem. Beer has the most carbs, about 10-14 grams. However the new light beers may be as low as 5 grams of carbs. Wine has 5-10 grams of carbs.

Alcohol tends to stop any fat burning while your body processes the alcohol. One drink a day may not be harmful, and many studies indicate that one glass of wine maybe beneficial. That is likely from the antioxidants that are in it, which you can just get from grape juice. Overall it would be best to limit alcohol use to one or two on the weekends only.

Calories-In
How to Limit Them

Here are some basic feedback mechanisms that can help you limit your food and calorie intake. They rely on your body's natural instincts. In a way, you "trick" your body, or *TRain your stomICK*, (bad spelling to make the acronym) into thinking it is full enough.

First Calorie Limiting TRICK: A Full Stomach

Normally, your body turns off its hunger drive when your stomach is full. However, most of us do not heed that signal, especially when the food smells so good, looks enticing, or is just sitting in front of us at the table. As a result, our stomachs get stretched out, and our brain no longer responds to the "stop eating I'm full" signals. How can you restore that feedback mechanism? You need to let the stomach shrink back down to its natural size. This will take time. To help, here are a few suggestions.

Fill your stomach with low calorie fillers. This is a calorie free way to turn off your hunger drive, and therefore not eat as much.

Water is a good filler. Experts recommend we drink eight glasses a day. It has no calories and makes you full. A good habit is to have a glass or bottle of water with you at all times. Water, by itself, can empty out of your stomach in 20-30 minutes.

Dr Tim's Top Ten Tips
8
Drink More Water
(tea too)

More Than Just Water: Other water sources are welcomed, too. They are still mostly water, and you still reap the same benefits, and maybe more, as long as they don't have the "bad" things in them: namely sugar. Sugar substitutes are better than sweet drinks, but they may increase your hunger drive. I recommend stevia because it is plant based.

- Tea is a great alternate to plain water. It is full of antioxidants. Hot or cold.
- Coffee, the drink with the highest levels of antioxidants.
- Lemon water has the added fruit antioxidant benefits of lemons.
- Juices (unsweet) have the fruit benefits without the calories. I enjoy sugar-free cranberry juice.
- Diet Sodas: They are mostly water, but do have the possible toxic harm from its other chemicals and may increase your appetite.

Fiber is an even better filler. It is not absorbed and when taken with water, it is a great no-calorie filler. Fiber stays in the stomach longer and makes you feel fuller, which turns off the hunger drive for a longer time.

Fiber also helps reduce the risk for heart disease, stroke, diabetes and cancer. We all need more fiber in our diet. 30 grams of fiber a day is recommended by all the major medical associations. Most of us get only 10 to 15 grams a day. Each fruit and vegetable has about 3 grams per serving. So, most of us need to supplement our fiber intake.

You can get the zero calorie fiber in powder form. Just a scooping in a glass of water before each meal can work wonders. They also come as fiber bars or fiber capsules, or even fiber gummies. High fiber cereals or oatmeal also make very good fillers, but they do have carbohydrate calories that you may want to limit. Fruits and vegetable are another good fibrous filler.

Dr Tim's Top Ten Tips
#9
Eat More Fiber.
Get all you can get.

Second Feedback TRICK: Eat Slowly.

When you are taking in calories, eat slowly to give your stomach time to fill up and send back the "full" message to the hunger drive center. This takes 10 to 30 minutes. That is one reason Europeans tend to weigh less. They spend the whole evening eating, yet they don't eat as much; perhaps they spend more time talking, leaving less time to put calories in their mouth. That is something we could try too. Another great way to slow down eating is to chew your food slowly and repeatedly. For example, count 20-30 chews for each bite of food you take.

Good Gum

Studies have found that simply chewing gum can decrease the hunger drive, letting you go longer without eating. The brain responds to the chewing as a feedback, thinking the body has received some food. Chewing every bite of food 30+ times has been associated with weight loss too. So chew away.

Third TRICK: Eat Frequent Small Meals.

Small meals keep you from getting hungry, yet allow the stomach to shrink. Insulin levels stabilize with small meals, and total calorie intake on average is less with small meals, which results in weight loss.

It can take a good four weeks or more for the stomach to shrink back to "normal" size, depending on how much you stretched it out. Once it is smaller, you will be amazed at how quickly you fill up. Hence, all the emphasis on "snacks" in stead of "meals."

Fourth TRICK: Eat High-Quality Foods

Eating quality foods is what this book is all about. It those high-fiber, high-antioxidant, low-trans fat foods we have discussed. They satisfy the body so you will eat less. For example, people who eat high-quality protein diets have been found to consume at least 10% less calories a day. People who eat quality carbohydrates (fruits and vegetables) eat less of the junky carb foods. People who consume olive oil eat less of the toxic trans fatty acid foods. What more can I say.

Well-rounded meals that include lean meat, vegetables, and fruit, can be satisfying and filling, without needing large amounts. The old fashion homemade meals, with all the starches (bread, potatoes) and desserts, just fill us with unneeded calories. That's fine if you are a growing kid, burning off the calories every day. But as the metabolism slows in adulthood, it is a habit that is time to break free of.

Meal replacements can be quality foods and can be an important part of a diet plan. They work nicely early on in a diet and can be bought in most groceries. The highest quality ones have all the elements your body could use. An example is Ensure. One can equals a meal. These are usually for ill folks having trouble eating. The diet meal replacements can work well, the higher protein ones in particular. They can come as a protein drink or protein bar, which could save you from eating a whole high calorie fast food meal. Packaged frozen diet meals can also help control your total calorie intake and be quite satisfying. And, the newer ones seem to taste better!

Fifth Feedback TRICK: Eat Less Carbs.

As discussed earlier, consuming less carbs reduces the insulin feedback mechanism that drives hunger. You have read about the ravages of a high carbohydrate diet: how carbs cause the crazy carb cycle, insulin resistance, metabolic syndrome, and ultimately diabetes and obesity. But how do you reduce those carbs when they are typically 60 percent of your diet? Once I see the warnings in the blood tests, I give patients a simple three steps to reduce their carbs. Of course, this also typically results in weight loss too.

Sugar Substitutes

Sugar substitutes may help people lose weight, but recent studies indicate people who drink diet drinks tend to gain weight. It is thought to be due to an increase in hunger drive because the body still releases some insulin thinking it is getting sugar, or people think they can eat more of the bad stuff, since they are drinking a diet drink. The substitutes can help with blood sugar control for diabetics, according to a joint statement issued by the AHA and ADA. Stevia is considered the safest of the sugar substitutes since it is plant-based.

Steps to Reducing Carbs and the Hunger Drive

1. No Sweet Drinks!

Wean yourself off the sweetened sodas and sweet teas. Based on the above explanation, there is no way you will break the carb cycle and lose weight if you don't get rid of those sweet drinks.

Most patients will claim that the diet drinks don't taste as good, and they are right. I found this true myself. But I challenge them, like I challenged myself: Go one month with no sweet drinks, and when you taste them again they will taste too sweet. It is truly just a matter of taste and what your taste buds are used to. It takes about a month to break a habit and change your tastes, hence the four-week plan.

2. Get ride of the sweets and snacks.

This includes the "low fat" snacks. The best thing is to just get them out of the house. These are the comfort foods that you will tend to give into in your weaker moments. If they are not in the house, they are less of a temptation.

Some people claim they have to have a piece of chocolate after a meal. One piece of chocolate, or a bite of desert, is not the problem. It is the whole candy bar after each meal, and between meals, or the bowl of ice cream you just gotta have every night that's trouble. Just one or two bites can satisfy that hunger craving. Unfortunately, it is not easy to stop with one or two bites.

3. Cut back on the starches.

Starches are bread, pasta, potatoes, and rice. For many, our weakness is either pasta or potatoes (including potato chips and French fries). Start by cutting your servings in half. Most of us pile up our plate with these starches, yet they are just cheap high carb fillers. Try taking a double serving of vegetables as your filler instead.

Most of us grew up with starches at every meal, especially supper. These are the old "staple" foods necessary in the farming days when you needed something to keep your energy up while working out it the fields. Those calories were quickly burned up. No one seems to be burning those kind of calories anymore.

Hungry? That's good!

That means you are burning fat. You will naturally feel hungry if you are loosing weight, your body will want more calories. Try to wait a little while if you feel hungry. But do not let the pangs get overwhelming or when you finally eat you then tend to over eat. That is why you should always eat just a little snack to keep the hunger pangs in control.

Calories-Out

Burn the Fat

Metabolism (metabolic rate): Metabolism is the energy used in living cells for all processes of life. The higher your metabolism the more energy (calories) you burn. Unfortunately, everything slows as we age, even our metabolism.

1. Maintain your metabolic rate. Just as a fire needs constant fuel to keep it burning, so does your body. If your body goes more than 12 hours without food, it starts to conserve energy by decreasing its metabolism. It slows down the fire. That's why it's important to eat small amounts throughout the day. Eat when you are hungry, but not too much. Keep your body supplied or it will start storing up the food as fat and therefore burn fewer calories. You risk accomplishing nothing by eating less. Worse than that, when your body finally gets food, it is more likely to store some of it because it doesn't know when more food will arrive.

2. Increase your metabolic rate: There is basically one safe way to burn excess calories: exercise.

Exercise. Though you may not like it, all successful weight management programs include exercise. A recent study found that exercise in the morning burns more fat than carbohydrates or proteins. Exercise is important, but it is something you need to start slowly with if you have not done much in the way of exercise. It does not necessarily need to involve going to the gym, and using weights. It can be a simple as walking. I will be discussing efficient ways to get the most out of that hard-earned fat burning activity.

Do Something

The NIH (National Institute of Health) spent thousands of our tax dollars studying exercise and its benefits. Here's what they found: **"Something is better than nothing,"** and, **"The more you do, the better off you are."** How's that for money well spent?

It is good to know that your body likes to be active, and the more active the better. So why aren't we exercising? As I mentioned earlier, our bodies are quite efficient when it comes to conserving energy. We naturally would rather sit than walk, and walk than run, etc. We are just being efficient. In essence, we're lazy in an efficient way. The bad thing is, this does not help you burn calories, which leads to fat and flabby bodies.

The word exercise brings a lot of different thoughts to mind. Many cringe at the thought. Some assume they have to go to the gym, meaning one more expense of the membership and new outfit. Others go out and buy the latest exercise equipment, never used except as a clothes rack. Let me put your mind at rest. Exercise here means one thing: be more active. That simply means:

burn more calories by doing more. So relax, the only exercise requirement in this plan is walking.

I have long been a proponent of walking. Hippocrates said, "Walking is man's best medicine." And now, every year, more studies are documenting the benefits of walking. For example, one study shows that women who walk three hours a week (that's just 30 minutes 6 days a week!) lose 7% of their belly fat in a year. Not only do you lose fat from walking, you also improve your general health and wellbeing. For example, people who walk at least 3 hours a week reduce their risk of death by more than 50%. That's about as straight forward as it can get on the benefits of walking.

Another study showed you burn more calories by standing instead of sitting. So why not try eating while you stand. Offices are starting to provide standing workstations to encourage healthy activity.

And yet another study of note has shown that you burn more fat the 24 hours after you exercise compared to just during exercise. That means, if you exercise in the morning, you spend the whole day and night burning more fat. So why not get moving?

Dr Tim's Top Ten Tips
#10
WALK.
Keep moving,
the more the better.

Top Ten Advantages of Exercise

1. Increases metabolism: Burns calories long after your workout.
2. Builds muscles that can burn more calories.
3. Uses fat for fuel, not muscle.
4. Lowers the body's insulin levels.
5. Curbs the appetite.
6. Strengthens heart, lungs, brain, and every part of your body.
7. Lowers cholesterol.
8. Anti-aging effects. You can reduce your biological age by up to ten years!
9. Releases endorphins that make you feel great.
10. Improves blood flow to all organs, and decreases risk of blood clots.

Exercise is best in the morning:
- It burns more fat, all day.
- It is easier to schedule.
- It gives you more energy for the day.

Exercise also has many mental benefits too:
- It improves concentration.
- It makes it easier to relax.
- It makes you feel better about yourself.
- It helps you sleep better at night.

Summary

By now you should have a basic understanding of the ingredients that are essential to any weight loss program. If you stop here, you should have learned enough to manage your own weight, as long as you're motivated to do so. Most people do better in a program with a friend or partner. Now I encourage you to continue reading as I explain the structure of this program and its simplicity.

Anti-Aging Diet

I will not go into detail on this lengthy subject matter. The Anti Aging fad is exploding with an unprecedented flood of confusing information. So, to keep it simple, I will summarize:

All the health benefit discussions so far in this book, can also apply to slowing the aging process. In particular: reducing inflammation and oxidation, by avoiding the bad fats and consuming more antioxidants from your fruits and vegetables and vitamins.

Furthermore, the total lifetime reduction of calories and increase in exercise has been associated with a longer life, not to mention the youthful skin benefits of fish oil, water, and antioxidants. Essentially, this book could also be considered an anti-aging book.

PART THREE
The Legitimate Diet
Weight Loss Plan

1. Drink more water.
- Helps you feel full.
- Flushes out toxins.
- Is good for your joints, muscles, skin, kidneys... your whole body.

2. Reduce the carbs. No sugar.
- Carbs often make up more than 60% of one's diet.
- Carbs are the highest source of useless calories.
- Eliminating carbs reduces your hunger drive.

3. Eat more protein, less fat.
- Protein is always a safe bet to eat.
- Protein is the main food your body does need.
- Protein builds muscle that burns fat and carbs.

4. Increase fiber intake
- Fiber keeps you full.
- Fiber helps you absorb less fat and lowers cholesterol.
- Fiber stabilizes sugar levels.

5. Exercise.
- Exercise builds muscle, which burns calories.
- Exercise promotes loss of fat.
- Exercise burns up the carbs.

How To Get Started

- Make the commitment to get started, and tell at least someone else. This will help hold you accountable. Better yet, do it with a friend, and hold each other accountable.
- Take the Legitimate Diet Test on the next page to see where you stand.
- Clean out the cupboard of the junk foods. Get rid of the snacks and bad carbs now before you give in. It's better to just throw it out than eat it. Think of it as cathartic. It proves your commitment.
- Stock up on your favorite protein: lean meats and lean protein snacks. They'll be handy when you are hungry and in a hurry. Get some protein powder and eggs.
- Stock up on fiber, good fruits and vegetables.
- See my Quick Start list in two pages, for more detail see my Top Ten Shopping List in the appendix.
- Get moving. Get a pedometer and start keeping track of your total steps each day. 10,000 steps is a good goal, which is almost 5 miles. You may be surprised how soon you get to 10,000 steps.
- Get ready to form good habits, and stop the old habits, and feel better for it. Your body may fight you, but hang in there, you can do it.

Diet Test

Here is a test to get you started. See where you stand now and where you need to improve. Get motivated, do the diet, and retest yourself. I am sure you will see improvement.
Instructions*: For each question write in the blank a number 1-7 for the best number that generally applies to you.*

1. How many hours do you watch TV per day? ___

2. How many hours of aerobic exercise per week? ___
   Walking or other exercise that increases your heart rate.

3. How many sweets or desserts per week? ___

4. How many servings of fruit per week? ___

5. How many servings of "junk food" per week? ___

6. How many servings of vegetables per week? ___

7. How many servings of red meat per week? ___

8. How many servings of fish or chicken per week? ___

9. How many times do you feel stressed per week? ___

10. How many vitamins do you take per day? ___

How to score:
- Add questions 2,4,6,8, and 10: Total Even ___
- Add question 1,3,5,7,and 9:   Total Odd ___
- Subtract the odd total from the even total for your score.

Your score: _____

- Poor: any negative number: You really need this diet.
- Weak: 0-10: Typical diet: Needs improvement.
- Not bad: 11-20: Your doing some things right. Work on it.
- Good: 20-30: Looking good. Just a few things to fix.
- Excellent: 30+: You've got the right diet going. Congrats.

Quick Start List

What I recommend as an easy start for this diet plan.
See my bigger shopping list in the appendix for more tips.

1. **Protein powder**: I use the blend I formulated, the ten best essential amino acids, pure and safe, and no additives.
2. A good **Multivitamin**: This will assure you get the nutrients and minerals you need, as you eat less foods.
3. Omega 3 **Fish oil**: Good healthy oils in a capsule, can help with satiety and benefits the brain and body as mentioned earlier. Get a safe pure brand.
4. **Fiber**: Powder is good, but I like fiber capsules, because they are easy to take any time. The perfect no calorie filler, goes well with water.
5. Fruit: **Berries**: are the lowest is carbs. **Blueberries** is what I would start with, they last a little longer, are easy to blend. **Raspberries** are my next favorite. **Apples** are easy to take with me, full of fiber, and last a long time. **Grapefruit** has been found to have enzymes that help promote fat burning.
6. Vegetables: Get a bunch of **celery** and **carrots**, (go great with dips) and a lot of **greens** (I like spinach or kale). **Green beans** (fresh or canned), **cucumbers and tomatoes**: these three are essentially calorie free, eat as much as you want.
7. Meat: Fresh **turkey**, chicken, canned **tuna** or sardines.
8. Drink: **water** (lots of water bottles), unsweet **tea**, and **coffee. Almond milk:** has no carbs, and is great for mixing protein powder or blending berries.
9. Snacks: **Nuts**, (almonds mainly, any will do), **Jerky**: turkey jerky is lower in fat and calories. **Protein bars**: I like the Adkins bars: they have zero carbs. **Pickles**: the non-sweet ones, at least with no added sugar.
10. Condiments: **mustard, black pepper** or other **peppers** and **hot sauces** add flavor plus they have been found to curb ones appetite. **Salt** can add flavor, is calorie free, but can fluid retention and raise BP, just don't use too much.

Fiber

As mentioned, fiber makes a great filler and it is not absorbed. It will keep your stomach full and your appetite satisfied longer on less calories.

- **Fiber powder:** It is the most basic form of fiber. It has no associated calories with it.
- **Fiber Capsules**. It takes a lot of capsules to fill you up. 6-8 capsules typically equal a scoop of fiber. It may be a lot of pills, but you don't taste the fiber.
- **Fruits and Vegetables** are also a great source of fiber, but carbs come with them. They help fill you up, so you should eat less total calories.
- **Breakfast Fibers:** Oatmeal is the best fiber cereal, and berries make good fiber fillers for breakfast.
- **Snack Fiber:** Fiber gummies make a great snack. Nuts, berries, apples, popcorn, and vegetables can also be a very good snack filler.

Top Ten Sources of Fiber

1. **Oatmeal**. Oatmeal is the best breakfast fiber source.
2. **Whole grains**. That means whole-wheat bread.
3. **Bran cereals.** Cereal with 5 grams of fiber or more.
4. **Berries**. Lower in carbs and great fiber source.
5. **Nuts**. Almonds, pecans, and walnuts have more fiber than other nuts.
6. **Apples:** It's the skin that's important here.
7. **Popcorn.** It's a great source of fiber.
8. **Brown rice.** White rice doesn't offer much fiber.
9. **Beans.** bean salad, bean burritos, chili, soup.
10. **Vegetables**. The crunchier, the better.

Protein

As discussed earlier, protein is going to be a great friend and essential component in your new diet plan.

- Protein supplies the nutrients you need (without the bad fat and carbs). Take a multivitamin too.
- Protein can fill you up, and satisfy your hunger with less calories (high quality food).
- High protein diets help lower cholesterol, diabetes, and heart risks.

Ten Best Low Calorie Protein Foods:

1. Fish. Especially, salmon, cod, mackerel, sardines, bass, and tuna.
2. Shellfish. Especially shrimp, crab, lobster, oysters, and scallops.
3. Eggs. Makes a great breakfast food, can be prepared many ways for variety.
4. Skim milk. Especially good with protein powder.
5. Soy. A common source for protein powders.
6. Turkey. The leanest of the white meats.
7. Chicken. A great standard, always available in restaurants when eating out.
8. Nuts. Walnuts, pecans, and almonds are the lowest in carbs. They all have the good fats.
9. Jerky. Make sure it is lean. There are a lot of good flavors now available. Makes a great snack.
10. Protein bars. A quick snack for weak hunger spells. Get the low carb bars.

Basic Day to Day Steps

The great thing about this diet is:
- You don't get too hungry.
- It takes advantage of your natural body mechanisms.
- If you do go off the diet, you can easily get back on it.

1. Exercise
Start with just a walk. Then gradually increase walking or try adding new exercises. Morning is the best time to exercise because you burn more fat in the morning especially if you exercise. If you simply cannot exercise in the morning, find a time that is best for your schedule. Remember, something is better than nothing. Even evening exercise, can be beneficial. Recent studies found that evening exercise it does not keep you awake, and people actually sleep better after good exercise.

2. Protein
Plan on using protein to replace carbohydrates and fat. For example, morning will be better to start the day with a protein powder drink, or eggs, fixed any way you like, instead of the usual cereal or toast. Later on, try protein power drink to replace other meals.

3. Fiber
Start with one serving or capsule a day, and increase to two a day in week 2, then three the third week. The fiber will fill your stomach so you will eat less. Fiber also has many health benefits.

4. Water
Drink a glass of water every chance you get. Ideally, you should drink eight 8 oz. glasses a day anyway, so start with two in the morning. Then keep a water bottle with you at all times, and sip it every chance you get.
Diet drinks are better than sweetened drinks, but not preferred because they might make you more hungry.

Top 10 Benefits of Water

1. Helps with weight loss: Water is calorie free and fills you up. And increases your metabolism and fat burning ability.
2. Maintains good fluid balance. Your body is 66% water.
3. Helps muscles work better. Improves energy transfer in muscles.
4. Helps keep your kidneys and other organs functioning well.
5. Helps flush out toxins. Water helps to neutralize oxidants.
6. Is nontoxic. Purified water does not have chemicals found in other drinks.
7. Maintains bowel function. Improves bowel elimination, including toxins.
8. Helps you look younger. Keeps your skin hydrated and healthy looking.
9. Helps with a good mood and better outlook.
10. Helps with pain. Water can reduce headaches and leg cramps.

The Approach to Each Meal

Breakfast

Burn your fat in the morning, and lose weight all day. Yep, morning is the best time to burn your fat. You've been fasting eight plus hours, and your body is ready to burn some fat, if it doesn't get a bunch of carbohydrates to stop it. So take advantage of that, and put your body to work burning that unwanted fat. You should eat breakfast, but make it low carb. Have a protein drink or eggs. Forget the toast, cereal, and pastries. Start your water intake early, and adding some fiber will help keep you full. Take a morning walk and you'll burn even more fat, throughout the whole day!

Lunch

Don't skip lunch. Remember, keep something in your stomach at all times, to maintain a steady metabolism. Salads make a great lunch. Lettuce or other greens act as a filler with limited calories. It is what you put on the lettuce that makes a difference. Low fat meat (like turkey or chicken) is permitted. A sandwich with fruit and or vegetable is good. Two slices of bread are acceptable, but limit the amount of bread to just that (or just throw away the bread). Wraps are also a good idea. They have less carbs than a sandwich, and can be filled with lots of healthy low carb choices of food. Even the fast food restaurants have jumped on this bandwagon, so being in a rush is not an excuse for eating poorly.

Afternoon Snack

If you have done well you may be hungry in the

afternoon. Do not give in to the quick carbohydrate fix. Other low calorie snacks are acceptable. Fruits or vegetables are best. You could consider protein bars. I recommend nuts as a snack because they have less carbs, healthy omega 3 fatty acids, and it doesn't take a lot to satisfy.

Dinner

If you have followed the plan so far, you are probably going to be hungry. You have earned a good meal. Enjoy. Take some fiber with water before you eat. Again, this will fill you up so you don't eat as much. And eat slowly! Go for more proteins and vegetables and less starches (potatoes and pasta and bread). This may take getting use to. At the end, you should feel full and satisfied. If you crave a dessert, try just a tiny serving (1-2oz) and savor it, for example one spoonful of ice-cream.

Evening Snack

If you are still hungry, try vegetables with a small amount of dip or some berries (they have less carbs). Eating in the evening is often done out of habit, perhaps while watching TV. Consider changing your habits. Try reading while sipping water or decaf tea. Better yet, take an evening stroll while your body is digesting. If this seems like too much work, don't worry at this point, you are learning a new habit and it can take time. Take it a day at a time.

That's it in a nutshell! Easy, right? A diet that is tolerable, simple, and lasts. If you are ready to give it a try, read on.

FOUR-WEEK PLAN
*It takes four weeks to break old habits
and start new habits.*

Week One

This first week is a transitional week. You will be learning new habits. Your body may resist the changes. It is critical to not give up. You probably will not lose a lot of weight this first week. It takes a little time for your body's metabolism and fuel burning to adjust. Most people make the mistake of trying to do it all the first day. They end up feeling starved and give in quickly because their body is demanding what it has been accustomed to.

Easy Exercise. In the morning, take a walk. If the weather is bad, go to the gym or find someplace indoors where you can walk around. This week start with just ten minutes if your body isn't used to walking.

Fiber. Take one serving or capsule with breakfast. This is the minimal amount and will not do much the first week, but it is important to start the habit. Also, most diets are so low in fiber that you might feel bloated if you take too much fiber at once. You should gradually increase the amount.

Protein. Let's start on some good protein too, try the powder in your cereal or oatmeal if you are not ready to give that up yet. Or try some eggs for breakfast instead of those high carb foods.

Water. Drink at least 3 glasses of water. Eliminate one sweetened drink each day. The most important thing is to stop the sweet drinks. Remember, you have to beat this habit before you'll lose any significant weight.

Breakfast. Begin the transition to more fruit and protein in the morning. Plan on less cereal, starch and sugar. Don't skip breakfast, which is easy to do. You need to eat something nutritious to keep that fire burning. Try some eggs or protein powder.

Lunch. Eat what you might normally eat this week, except drink just water or unsweet tea. Diet soda is ok for now, but ultimately you may want to give that up, since it could drive your hunger.

Mid Afternoon. This is a common time when unhealthy snacking occurs. Make note of what you are craving. Keep unhealthy snacks (candy, cookies, chips, etc.) out of sight. Instead, have an orange, apple, carrots, or nuts.

Supper. Take note of what you eat. Especially the amount of starches (bread, pasta, and potatoes) you tend to eat. Think about how you can start cutting down on the portions.

Evening. This is the other weak point of the day. Make note of what you tend to snack at night. TV is a common source of hunger stimulation. Try turning the television off, change the channel, or speed though commercials in DVR recorded shows.

Week Two

Now it is time to get more serious. This second week can be a challenge because you are starting to change some habits. Your body will want to stick with the old habits, but it's critical for you to stay with the program. Even a few bad days are better than seven bad days.

Exercise. Hopefully you established your baseline for each exercise. Try to add another 10 minutes to each exercise.

Fiber. Get into the habit of taking some fiber before ate least two meals per day.

Water. Try to add an extra glass of water each day this week. Water is much better than diet soda. It is time for sweetened drinks to go away.

Protein. If you have the powder, try it in the morning with some almond milk (has no carbs) or blend it with berries to make a shake. Could be used to replace any meal. Start experimenting with different combinations.

Breakfast. Start eating protein or eggs in the morning. It will stick with you longer and you should be less hungry by lunch. If you desire some sweetness, opt for berries or berry protein drink, instead of cereal or toast.

Lunch. Try a salad or sandwich. Lean meat and

condiments is fine on the sandwich. Each slice of bread is about 14g carbohydrates and 80 calories or more. If you do opt for bread, choose the high fiber or a wrap variety if you have a choice. Forget the chips.

Mid-afternoon. Craving may be most intense at this time of day. So have a low carbohydrate snack ready. Preferably, I know you've heard it before, fruits or vegetables. Otherwise high protein snacks are great, like peanuts, cheese, or protein bars. Sip on a cup of hot tea.

Dinner. You have earned a good meal. Enjoy! Eat slowly and make sure you're full and satisfied. Remember, choose more protein and vegetable dishes, and less starches such as potatoes and pasta.

Evening. You should not be hungry in the evening if you ate enough for dinner. If you are hungry, try vegetables with a small amount of dip or a protein bar. Also, drink your quota of water.

Fruit

Most people like fruit. Sometimes you may get tired of the same thing or forget to restock at the grocery. Go to the grocery weekly (never on an empty stomach), and try some different types of fruit. You really can't go wrong with any fruit. But the yellow fruits (bananas and pears, and watermelon) tend to have more carbs. Low carbohydrate fruits are raspberries, strawberries, and kiwi. The fructose in fruits does not affect sugar levels as much as other glucose containing foods.

Week Three

- This is the big week when your body should finally be adjusting to your lower calories and your hunger drive should be reduced.
- Your habits should be changing.
- You will see a pattern of your weak areas by filling out the daily chart.
- Hang in there. Establishing new habits requires patience. It takes about a month for a new habit to stick.
- You can relax on your diet this weekend, but you should eat less because your stomach is shrinking.
- If you are not achieving any weight loss, seriously and honestly evaluate what you are doing or not doing.

Exercise. You should have gotten in at least three days of good exercise. If you did, try intensifying this week. If you are walking 30 minutes at a gentle pace, increase the pace for ten minutes. Exercise tips the scales towards burning fat instead of muscle. The more the better.

Fiber. Now comes the challenge of fiber before every meal. That is the ideal, but if you can't do it, at least make sure it's twice a day, every day.

Protein. If you haven't already, make protein a regular staple. By now you should have tried a variety of options to use it. Half a scoop with water can make a nice before meal filler, or chose a meal to replace.

Water. Water helps increase your metabolism, and actually burn more fat, the more the better then. This week you should be drinking 7- 8 glasses of water a day.

Flushing It Out

Drinking more water results in an increase in urination, which in turn flushes out toxins. Some toxins are stored in fat, so as you break down the fat while losing weight, the toxins are released into the body's circulation. The kidneys filter these toxins. Water helps flush them out.

Breakfast. Try some eggs a different way, or stick with your protein drink. If you must have a cereal, oatmeal could be eaten. And feel free to enjoy some berries or other fruit: except no bananas.

Lunch. Instead of salads you may try different types of meat: turkey, grilled chicken, or fish are best. Cottage cheese, or any cheese, is a nice low carbohydrate choice. Peanut butter makes a good filler too, and has limited carbs per serving. But not any jelly, or just as smidgen.

Dinner. This is a meal to be enjoyed. Cravings should be decreasing. You should be satisfied sooner. Now it's time to think more about this meal. As mentioned, steer away from the worse carbohydrates: starches (potatoes, bread, and pasta). Go more for meats and vegetables. Have one slice of bread at the most. It is time to seriously cut back on the carbohydrates now. If you haven't lost much weight so far this could be why.

Evening. This still seems to be the downfall for most. I think we eat more out of habit or boredom at this time of day. So the best thing would be to change your habits, especially if you are watching TV. Try reading a book in a different room, or start a hobby. If you are busy, you are less likely to eat. If you are hungry, try vegetables with a small amount of dip.

If you're struggling:
- You should start to see where your weaknesses are, so work on one or two of them. Remember that you are developing a new habit, and it can take time.
- Call a friend who knows you, or has been through this.
- Be honest with yourself and take it a day at a time.
- Record at the end of the day what you ate, and note the times when you were hungry.
- Think of "feeling hungry" as a good thing: that means your burning fat. Just don't go too long being hungry, or you end up eating even more. That is why small healthy snacks are an important part of weight loss.

Nuts
Nuts of any type are excellent choices for meals or snack, although nuts do have as much carbohydrate as protein. The greatest benefit of nuts is their high polyunsaturated oil content. These oils have been found to reduce the risk for heart disease and promote healthy arteries. Good choices are walnuts, pecans, and almonds. The protein and fat will give more satisfaction than just carbs. They are high in calories though, so limit them to just a small handful, and savor them.

Take a break!

This is the end of the third week, the end of two intense weeks after the first transition week. This is when you get to take a break. No matter how much you have lost, you've earned two days off. Just forget about the diet. Enjoy.

You should find you fill up sooner than you would have three weeks ago, and you may not have as many cravings for junk food as you thought.

Every two weeks it is okay to take two days off from your diet. This gives your body a chance to readjust. If you have lost more than ten pounds, your body may try harder to conserve its fat. The two-day break lessens the body's conservation mechanism.

Meal Replacement Drinks

Meal Replacement Drinks can be a quality alternative for lunch. They provide the "quality" food you need to efficiently burn calories and remain satisfied. Most contain all 3 food types. The better ones for weight loss are high in protein, and lower in carbohydrate. In particular, a pure protein drinks make a better meal replacement when it comes to weight loss.

Week Four

You are rounding the corner for a healthier life. By now you are on your way to losing the weight you always wanted to. Plus, you have gained some excellent eating habits. Continue to develop your new eating habits. Exercise, fiber, and water should be a routine by now. Work on improving areas identified in your daily chart. It should really be taking hold now. If not, reassess your motivation. Look for things you've used as excuses.

Breakfast. Hopefully your new routine is water (or coffee or tea), with fiber capsules, and protein drink alternating with eggs and some berries. Remember, breakfast really is the most important meal. It sets your body's metabolism for the day.

Lunch. Instead of salads or meats you could consider protein bars or nutritional shakes. Or work in some low calorie soups: vegetable soup is ideal. Caned soup is ok, or make a big batch of soup to last all week, or freeze some for later.

Dinner. If the meals are getting monotonous, check out the low carbohydrate recipes in popular magazines. Or buy a low carb cookbook. Dinner is traditionally the biggest meal but it does not have to be. If you had a good lunch, try eating smaller portions for supper.

Congratulations, you have completed the course!

- It wasn't so bad, was it? As a matter of fact, wasn't it the easiest diet that really works?

- You can always continue what you started. If you go off the diet (perhaps if you go on vacation), you can easily resume it.

- If weight loss slows down or stops, don't worry. This is common after the first 15 to 20 pounds. The body is just trying to protect itself. You may want to increase your exercise regimen or change it to avoid boredom.

- It you want a more intense weight loss regimen, you can consider the Low Carb Diet described below.

Low Carb Diet Option

This is a more extreme diet for those who want a jump-start, or require a quick early response. It takes more discipline and commitment. In this diet, you reduce your total carbohydrate (carb) intake to less than 60g, or in the extreme, less than 30g. That allows 10g to 20g per meal, a very limited amount. You will need to read labels carefully. It is rather simple otherwise. Make up the calories with whatever fat and protein you like.

How a Low Carb Diet Works

There are many books with theories on how this works. Here are the basic principles:

- Eliminating carbs eliminates a significant energy supply. Remember that excess energy is stored as fat.
- It is difficult to make up the 50-60% of carbs a day you normally eat with fat and protein. But you can have fun trying.
- If you don't have the carbs to burn, your body will find something else to burn, such as the protein or fat you eat, and the fat you have stored up.
- It's easier to burn carbs than fat and protein. Your body will resist at first, but as long as it isn't given significant carb fuel, it will burn the fat.
- It takes more energy to burn fat and protein, and the breakdown produces some waste, so you need to drink more fluid to flush this out.
- Exercise is still important to avoid muscle break down.
- It is important to keep your stomach supplied with fat and protein because they burn slower. You need a steady supply to maintain the energy needs of the body.
- Carbs are allowed in limited quantities. Vegetables are the preferred source.
- Do not go below 30 carbs. No advantage has been found for going less than 30 carbs per day.
- Take a multivitamin to replenish any nutrients you may lose.
- Continue your fiber intake. It is not absorbed and it

can prevent constipation that sometimes goes along with this diet.

- After two weeks, you can gradually increase carbohydrate intake with fruits and vegetables, but still NO STARCHES (bread, pasta, and potatoes). Increase by 20g of carbohydrate each week. Don't go over 100g of carbs a day.
- Your cholesterol levels may increase initially, but after a month it will stabilize and then decrease.

Reduced Insulin Levels

Another advantage of limiting your carbs is that you also limit the amount of insulin needed. This eliminates the sugar ups and downs, which stops the yo-yo cravings previously mentioned. This also decreases after-meal fatigue and increases energy. Furthermore, insulin causes water retention, so less insulin causes more urine output, resulting in a quick loss of up to five pounds of fluid.

It takes several days for the body to adjust from burning carbs, to burning fat, which are two very different metabolic processes. The first week's challenge is to limit the carbs and force the body to lower its glycemic stores. It will adjust and burn fat as long as you don't throw too many carbs its way (less than sixty a day). Discipline is critical. I do not recommend a back and forth process from the extreme low carb diet to a lot of carbs.

For my easy low carbohydrate diet version see below. This is what I tell all my patients with any elevation in their glucose or insulin levels, especially diabetics.

Three Steps to Giving Up the Carbs

1. First, and most important: Stop drinking sweet drinks. If you do nothing else, you have to stop sweet drinks this week. Sweet drinks are like pouring the sugar right into you blood stream since it is absorbed so fast. There is no way you will loose weight unless you stop.

Note: Alcohol counts as a sweet drink. One drink per day may not be harmful, but it turns off any fat burning you are doing.

2. Stop the snacks and sweets. This seems obvious. But this also includes popcorn and pretzels. They are low in fat, but that just means they have more carbs.

3. Finally, reduce the starches: bread, pasta, potatoes, and rice. The old fashion habit of starch with every meal needs to become a thing of the past. Replace the starch servings with vegetables.

Apple Diet

A simple diet. You eat half of an apple before each meal and you eat less. It works! Try a half apple or grapefruit before each meal for a change of pace.

Diet Alternatives

Fasting Diets: A newer diet that has been found to work is essentially fasting one or two days a week. What they do: pick one or two days a week to eat no more than five hundred calories that day, it's easier to get through because you know it is only one day, and the next day you can eat normal again. It turns out, most people don't gorge themselves enough the next day to make up for the calorie loss the day before.

As far as a legitimate diet, I think it is a reasonable short-term alternative for a week or two to try the "fast for a day". This can be especially helpful if you are stuck or plateaued at your current weight, in spite of adhering to a good diet.

Vegetarian Diets: Have been around along time, allow too much carbs: flour and sugar. But recently there are new takes on them. Pescetarian Diet; a vegetarian diet that include seafood. Seems to offer lots of health benefits: fruits in AM, vegetables in PM, and seafood daily. Then there is the Paleo Diet that goes back to the hunter gatherer days. And there is the Fork over Knives Film and diet that is even more plant based. All make good points in a faddish way.

The Mediterranean diet: has a lot of variations and a lot of physician support, has good healthy choices, but limited in weight loss benefits. Overall, I think the Legitimate Diet is the best diet because it pulls all the best science together, with the easiest methods that put your body to work for you, naturally.

Soup Diets

There have been many soup diets through the years, the best known maybe the cabbage soup diet, which works, but only tolerable for about one week. Other soup diets can work great for a time, mixing it up works better.

How soup helps you lose weight

- Soup is more filling because of its water content. Studies have shown that soup keep us full longer than 'dry' foods.
- Soups are a great way to cut down on refined carbohydrates like bread or pasta. You don't really need crackers or bread to enjoy a hearty soup.
- Soup is packed with nutrients. Vegetable based soups are an excellent source of nutrients and soluble fiber. It is easy to add good quality protein to soup, like chicken, salmon or tofu. And, soups are naturally low in fat.
- The heat and water helps increase metabolism for more fat burning. Adding spices can help too.
- Avoid the creamy, high fat soups. Read labels before you buy.

I recommend trying some healthy soups as a meal alternative throughout your legitimate diet process.

References: Some of what I have read the past twenty years.
- Web MD: An excellent resource with many good articles. I recommend them for further advice and research.
- Multiple articles read from American Diabetic Association, American Medical Association, Archives of Internal Medicine, American Journal of Cardiology, Annals of Internal Medicine, Center For Disease Control, and National Institute of Health.
- Books: "Heart Attack Proof" by Michael Ozner, "Top Zone Foods", by Barry Spears, Ph.D., "The Carbohydrate Addict's LifeSpan Program" by Drs Richard and Rachael Heller, "Protein Power" M and M Eads, MD, "Wheat Belly" by William Davis, "Mayo Clinic Diet" by Mayo Clinic, "South Beach Diet" by Arthur Agatston

APPENDIX

Protein Bars are ideal choices for between meal snacks (which will be worse early in the diet while your body adjusts to your new regimen). It will ultimately be more satisfying to your body than candy bars, cookies, etc. It is very important to look at the amount of carbohydrates in the bars. Many bars say they are "protein bars," yet they still have 20-30 g of carbohydrates. This may be okay because you are getting all three food types, but if you are on the low carb diet, pay close attention.

Feel free to eat a protein bar whenever you feel hungry.

What about Diet Supplements? Supplements, or weight loss pills, typically claim to "curb your appetite" or "burn the fat." There are many different types out there. Some are actually dangerous. The well known ones (Ma Huang or Ephedra) can raise your blood pressure, cause palpitations, and increase anxiety. These may be able to curb your appetite for a few weeks, but then do nothing as your body gets use to them. Overall, the risks outweigh the benefits. They are not worth it.

Diet drinks and sugar-free candies require caution. Sugar-free may mean no carbohydrates, but saccharine or aspartame are replacing the sugars. These ingredients may increase the insulin levels, which in turn stimulates your hunger drive. Minimize these.

Stress and Dieting

Stress can affect your ability to lose weight. Stress raises cortisol levels, which tend to increase insulin levels, resulting in resistance to weight loss, and possible weight gain. Some people tend to eat more when stressed. Although stress is a part of our lives, perhaps this is a good time for you to look at how you are dealing with it.

- Take some quiet time for yourself; you would be amazed at what a five-minute break can do.

- Try deep, slow breathing. It too can be quite relaxing.

- Play music, games, or do that favorite activity you haven't had time for lately.

- Turn off the TV: Don't watch bad news, it makes you more anxious and depressed.

- Keep a diary of your stressors, how you deal with them, and what you ate when stressed. It can be quite revealing, and help relieve your stress too.

- Increase aerobic exercise. It is a diversion, which helps reduce stress. A brisk walk can work out that anxious energy while burning calories.

Carbohydrates in Foods

Carbohydrates grams per serving. Those in bold are better for you.

FRUIT				
Apple	18		Pasta	28
Banana	25		Pizza(slice)	20
Blackberries	**12**		Rice	32
Blueberries	**14**		Stuffing 40	
Cantaloupe	12			
Cherries	20		**VEGETABLES**	
Cranberries	12		Beans	18
Fruit Cocktail	32		**Broccoli**	**2**
Grapefruit	**15**		**Cabbage**	**4**
Grapes	16		Carrots	9
Kiwi	9		**Celery**	**1**
Orange	12		Coleslaw	15
Peach	12		Corn	24
Pair	20		Cucumber	6
Pineapple	17		Green beans	7
Plum	9		**Lettuce 0**	
Raisins	30		**Mushroom**	**2**
Raspberries	**8**		Onion	12
Strawberries	**8**		Potatoes	30
Tangerine	9		French fries	30
Watermelon	30		**Radish**	**1**
			Spinach	**3**
			Tomato	**6-8**

BREAD, CEREAL, GRAIN				
Bagel	28		**OTHER**	
Bread (slice)	14		**Nuts**	**8 (1oz)**
Bun	20		**Meats**	**0**
Cereal	20-30		**includes fish and poultry**	
Cookie(1oz)	20-30 each			
Chips	20-30		**Cheeses**	**0**
Crackers	28		**Eggs (2)**	**0**
Muffins	28		**Tofu**	**0**
Oatmeal28				
Pancakes	30			

Exercising
Aerobic Exercises

Walking is simply the best all-around exercise.
- Easy, no training, natural.
- 30 minutes each day (or 3 hours a week) at least.
- Improves lung function and brain blood flow.
- Can be done anytime. Mornings are best.
- Can be done anywhere, like at work during a lunch break.
- Builds abdominal muscles, reducing abdominal fat and waist size.
- Improves back muscle strain and pain.
- Listen to music using headphones to make it more enjoyable and relaxing.
- Speed up in the middle of your routine for more benefit.
- Wear quality shoes that are less than a year old.
- You could invest in a pedometer, or one of the new fitness wristbands. Set a goal of 2000 to 10,000 steps a day. It can add to you motivation.
- I round out about 2000 steps to a mile.

Relaxing Exercises
Average Calories Burned per Hour

Low Level	*High Level*
Slow walk (2 mph): 120 cal/hr,	JOG (6 mph): 360 cal/hr,
Brisk walk (4 mph): 240 cal/hr	Run (8 mph): 480 cal/hr
Bicycle (8 mph): 120 cal/hr	Bicycle (15 mph): 300 cal/hr
Gardening: 150 cal/hr	Swimming: 300 cal/hr
Golf: 150 cal/hr	Tennis: 225 cal/hr

Easy Indoor Exercises

Studies have shown that muscle-building exercises may help you lose weight faster. They can also strengthen your bones. You do not need weights to build muscle.

1. Push Ups: Build upper body, improves posture, uses <u>all</u> your muscles

2. Sit Ups: It firms your abdomen (but wont remove fat any faster from your belly, only total loss of fat will do that) and helps back pain. How to do sit ups: Lay flat on the floor on your back, knees bent. Slide hands from thighs up to knees, while raising shoulders off the floor slightly, then back down, a repeat 20+ times.

3. Jumping Jacks: quick leg muscle work out if you don't have the time to walk. Help loosen up tight muscles and joints. The deeper the knee bend, the more the benefit.

4. **Lunges/Knee Bends**: Step and bend forward on one leg while stooping down and hold as long as you can, then back up, and use the other leg. Repeat.

5. **Stair Climbing**: If it's a rainy day, just go up and down a flight of stairs 20 times.

Food Choices

	Choose	Avoid
Meat/Protein	Lean cuts of meat, chicken or turkey white meat without skin, fish: any kind including shellfish, tofu, sushi, eggs	Beef, pork, lamb, liver, sausage, bacon, lunchmeat, hot dogs
Dairy Products	Skim milk, Greek yogurt, cottage cheese, cheese with less than 4 grams of fat	Whole milk, cream, sour cream, cream cheese, hard cheeses (Swiss, American, cheddar)
Fats and Oils	Corn, olive, peanut, canola, safflower, soybean oils. Nuts, seeds, avocadoes, and olives, vinegar and oil	Butter, lard, bacon fat, coconut oil, palm oil, cheesy or creamy sauces or dressings
Grains: Bread and Cereals.	Multigrain breads, high fiber cereals, oatmeal, high fiber spaghetti, black rice	Sweet rolls, doughnuts, croissants, danish, pancakes, muffins, white bread, bagels, pasta, white rice
Fruits and Vegetables	Most fruits and vegetables, especially berries and dark green vegies, black beans	Potatoes, watermelon, bananas, pears, raisins, fruit cocktail
Snacks	Nuts, sugar free popsicles or sherbet, protein bars (low carb), unbuttered popcorn, pickles, dried fruit or vegetable chips	Cookies, candy, cakes, pies, ice cream, potato chips, corn chips, crackers, pizza
Drinks	Water, coffee, tea, sugar free juices, diet sodas	Whole milk, milkshakes, Frappuccino, juices, regular sodas

Dr. Tim's Top Ten Lists

Healthy Shopping List

1. **Strategy**: Eat before you go, never shop hungry. Prepare a list to avoid impulse buying. Shop in the outer isles, along the periphery, that's where you tend to find the healthier natural foods. The main isles tend to have the processed foods.

2. **Meat Dept**: canned tuna or sardines,sliced smoked turkey from the deli, fresh chicken breast, salmon, any other seafood. Tofu.

3. **Dairy Dept**: fresh eggs, skim milk, fat free ranch dip, cottage cheese, Feta cheese, low fat cheese, Parmesan cheese, Greek yogurt.

4. **Vegetable Dept**: broccoli, cauliflower, carrots, celery, salad mix , spinach, radishes, beans, cucumbers, mushrooms, tomatoes, tomato sauce (low sugar). Pretty much any vegetable. Fresh is preferred, but frozen can be as nutritious. Eat with dips or use for cooking. Mix and match to whatever your preference. Vegetables are what will fill you up, replace the garbage foods, and are the staples for your healthy life and weight lost. So buy up.

5. **Fruit Dept**: Berries, apples, grapes, grapefruit, and any other fruit on sale. Avoid the bananas and watermelons.

6. **Breads/Grains**: Multi grain bread (thin sliced), very high fiber cereal, oatmeal, low fat popcorn, Quinoa, brown rice, high fiber pasta.

7. **Nuts/olives/pickles**: walnuts, pecans, pistachios, almonds. Fresh or canned. Olives and pickles: any type, just not with added sugar. There are a lot of new gourmet styles.

8. **Liquids: Drinks and Oils**: a jar of olive oil and safflower oil for hotter cooking, and a jar of vinegar for cooking, Balsamic vinaigrette dressing, or other oil/vinegar dressings. Water, sugar-free cranberry juice, other sugar-free drinks, coffee, tea.

9. **Herbs and spices:** (fresh and dried) anything to spice up the meal: mustard, pepper, salt, chili powder, ginger, cinnamon, basal.

10. **Desserts**: sugar free sherbet and popsicles, dark chocolate that is at least 70 cocoa, chocolate protein bars, light whipped cream to put on berries.

Dr. Tim's Top Ten Tips
Eating Out Tips

1. Eat something before you go out so you're not so hungry and you order less.
2. Minimize alcohol (extra calories, has carbs, and reduces diet self-control).
3. Order a salad.
4. If marked on the menu, order the heart healthy meals.
5. Order grilled fish, other seafood, or turkey. But not fried.
6. Order a healthy appetizer as your main course.
7. Avoid the fried foods (the grease is a lot of extra calories).
8. Choose a baked potato over french fries or steak fries.
9. Order double the vegetables instead of potatoes or other starches.
10. Eat half (take the rest home for later).

Dr. Tim's Top Ten Tips
For Fast Food

1. Salads: There is quite a variety to choose from.

2. Soups: If they're not cream-based, they can be low cal. Soups and salad deals are great.

3. Chicken sandwich (grilled, not deep fried).

4. No french fries (about 10 calories per fry).

5. Chili is ok if it has beans (less fat in it).

6. Pizza: Get the thin crust and eat only one slice, with vegetables on top.

7. Chinese: Tofu or vegetables, no rice.

8. Japanese: sushi is very low fat.

9. Mexican: Chicken or beef fajitas or taco salad.

10. The grocery or food stores: Most of themn now have a salad and soup bar to go. This could be your best option for healthy fast food diet.

Dr. Tim's Top Ten Tips
Low Carb Meal Tips

1. Cheeses are great! Better if they are low fat. There are lots of varieties to try. There are protein crackers now that you could have with them.
2. Dips are low carb and go well with anything. Protein crackers or chips could work, or use vegetables (celery or carrots).
3. Eggs and turkey bacon make a great breakfast, add lean cheese and you've got an omelet. Try other meats for a variety, like crab or shrimp.
4. Condiments are generally okay, but limit the ketchup and barbecue sauce which have a fair amount of carbs. Feel free to enjoy salt and pepper and other spices.
5. Seafood of any type is a great choice, but avoid deep fried food.
6. Salads are always a good option. You can add generous amounts of low fat cheese or meat, nuts, other vegetables. Try vinegar or oil dressings. *Do not use low fat dressing because it is mostly carbohydrate.*
7. Vegetables such as spinach, lettuce, radishes, and alfalfa sprouts, broccoli and cauliflower are lowest in carbs. Its nearly impossible to get too many carbs from vegetables. You will be full before that happens.
8. Nuts are high in protein and fat, but have about 8 grams of carbs per serving. Eat small amounts. They make a great snack. Pickles are considered carbs and calorie neutral, and makes a great snack.
9. Increase fluids, water with lemon, tea, always unsweetened. Avoid diet sodas as they may still make you hungry.
10. Protein Bars make an excellent snack too. They can satisfy that mid day sweet tooth craving.

Dr. Tim's Top Ten Tips
Healthy Substitution Tips

1. Bean flour can be substituted in place of all-purpose flour. A quarter cup of fava or white bean flour has 8 grams of fiber, plus protein, minerals, and antioxidants, compared to the nutritionally depleted flour.
2. Frozen fruit can be used instead of jam. They have half the calories, with Vitamin C, fiber, and antioxidants. They taste great if warmed with cinnamon or ginger.
3. Avocado can replace butter. Use half a tablespoon of avocado for every tablespoon of butter in baked goods like brownies and cupcakes. You could spread it on toast or crackers. It can save 75 calories and replaces the saturated fat with the good unsaturated fats.
4. Hummus can substitute mayo. Hummus can be used as a sandwich spread, and in some sauces. It saves 65 calories per tablespoon and provides fiber, protein, and iron.
5. Greek yogurt can be used instead of sour cream, cream cheese, or mayo dips. For example, I've had a great yogurt spinach and kale. You save 60 calories per tablespoon and eliminate the trans fats. Greek yogurt with fruit can rival ice cream for desert with even more calorie and trans fat reduction.
6. Applesauce substituted for oil, butter, or sugar. A well-known baking substitute.
7. Rolled oats can replace breadcrumbs in recipes.
8. Baked or broiled broccoli or other vegetables can be as tasty and crunchy as baked fries or chips.
9. Turkey (ground) could replace any ground beef or sausage recipe.
10. Quinoa for rice ads 60% protein and reduces calories by 15%.

Dr. Tim's Top Ten Tips
How To Read Nutrition Labels

It is very helpful to understand nutrition labels. Don't be threatened by them. Labels provide helpful information about carbs, fats, and protein. It's most helpful for you to see how many carbs are really in the foods you eat. You may be surprised. I recommend making a habit of reading every label of the foods you buy, just to get a feel for what you are really eating.

1. Note the serving size. It is usually smaller than what you would normally eat.

2. Note serving per container. You can typically eat more than one serving at a time, so you have to multiply the calories by how many serving.

3. Note the total calories (that is what ultimately matters in losing weight).

Nutrition Facts

Serving Size 4oz
Serving Per Container 5

Amount Per Serving

Calories 100

	% Daily Values*
Total Fat 5g	**8%**
Saturated Fat 3g	**15%**
Trans Fat 1g	
Sodium 30mg	**1%**
Total Carbohydrate 30g	**10%**
Dietary Fiber 5g	**20%**
Sugars 15g	
Protein 8g	**16%**

* Percent Daily Values are based on a 2,000 calorie diet.

4. Note the fat label, the only concern would be to avoid the trans fatty acids and saturated fats.

5. Most importantly, read the total carbs.

6. You can subtract out the fiber from the total carbs.

7. You can also subtract out a dietary sugar that is not absorbed which is listed as sugar alcohol, e.g. maltose, found in diet protein bars.

8. The amount of sugar listed is straight forward, and is best if under 10 grams.

9. Total carbs minus the fiber and sugar leaves the starch in the food. Starch is a carb to be avoided, and best if under 15 grams.

10. Protein is good. Try to buy items with more protein than carbs.

Doctor Tim's Top Ten Tips
To Good Healthy Eating

#1: Eat less white stuff. Eat two less servings of the white stuff (refined flour and sugar) each day.

#2: Eat more fruit. Have an extra fruit and vegie each day.

#3: Eat less red meat. Give up the red meats. No more than one serving a week.

#4: Eat more fish. Or oil. Have a serving of seafood or fish oil everyday.

#5: Eat more nuts. A great crunchy snack.

#6: Eat more eggs. Don't worry about the yolk.

#7: Take a multivitamin with minerals daily.

#8: Drink more water, and tea too.

#9: Eat more fiber. Any way you can get it.

#10: Just Walk. Keep moving.

Made in the USA
Middletown, DE
01 February 2018